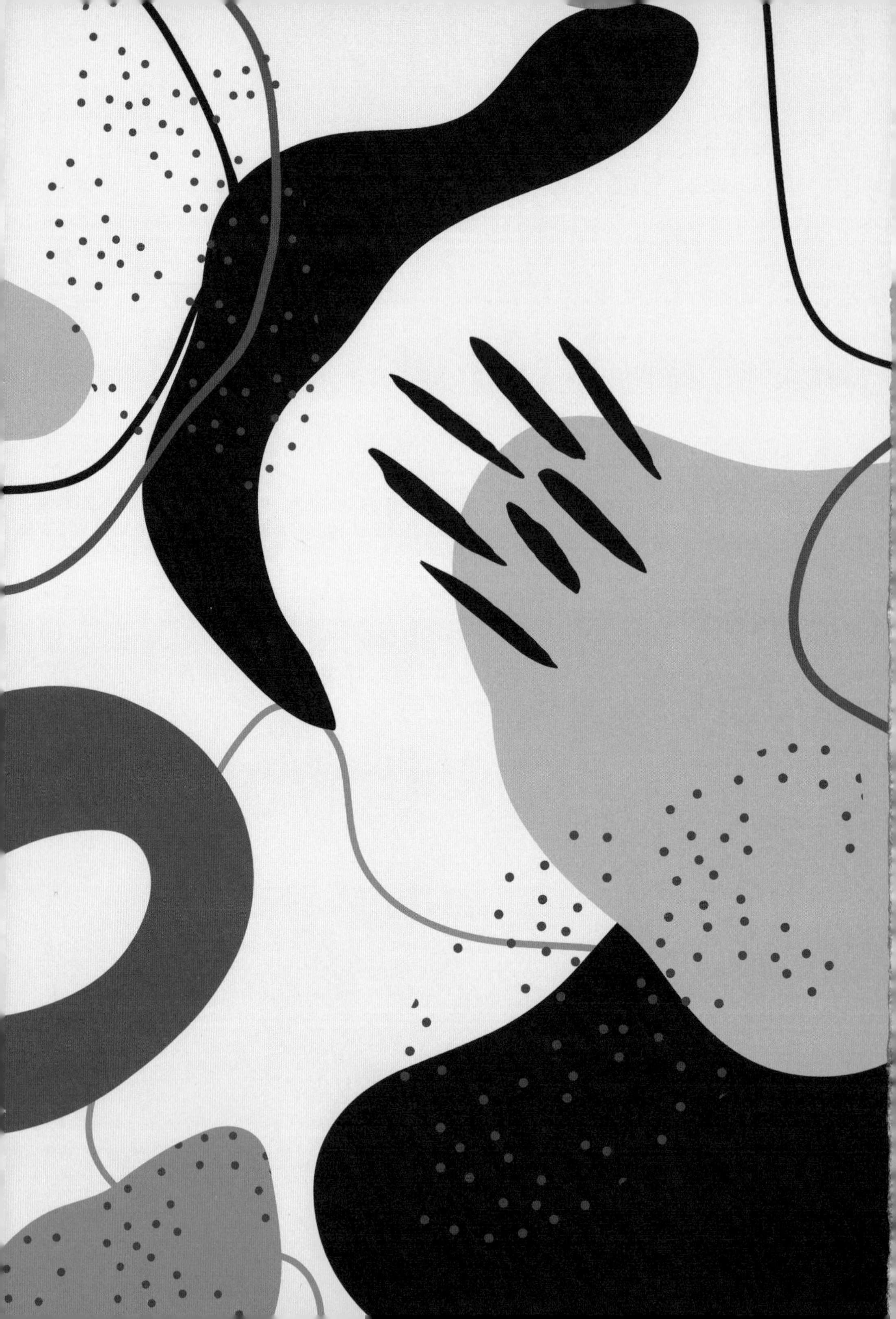

The Empowerment Cycle